53 Hair Loss Juice Recipe Solutions:

Juice Your Way to Healthier and Stronger Hair Using Natures Ingredients

By

Joe Correa CSN

COPYRIGHT

ACKNOWLEDGEMENTS

This book is dedicated to my friends and family that have had mild or serious illnesses so that you may find a solution and make the necessary changes in your life.

53 Hair Loss Juice Recipe Solutions:

Juice Your Way to Healthier and Stronger Hair Using Natures Ingredients

By

Joe Correa CSN

CONTENTS

ABOUT THE AUTHOR

After years of Research, I honestly believe in the positive effects that proper nutrition can have over the body and mind. My knowledge and experience has helped me live healthier throughout the years and which I have shared with family and friends. The more you know about eating and drinking healthier, the sooner you will want to change your life and eating habits.

Nutrition is a key part in the process of being healthy and living longer so get started today. The first step is the most important and the most significant.

INTRODUCTION

53 Hair Loss Juice Recipe Solutions: Juice Your Way to Healthier and Stronger Hair Using Natures Ingredients

By Joe Correa CSN

Having beautiful and healthy hair is something special. Our hair, like everything else in our body, is a living organism that has its own natural cycle of growth. This cycle has three phases – anagen, catagen, and telogen phase. Each phase is important. Most hairs on your scalp are in their anagen phase or a growth phase. This phase lasts from two to eight years and depends on many different factors. The other two phases include a transition and a resting period. Most people lose about 50 to 100 strands of hair each day. This is considered normal and nothing to worry about.

You have to keep in mind that your hair reflects your overall health condition. It is crucial to fill your diet with proven hair growth nutrients and to improve your health from within. One of the first superfoods you should consume in order to prevent hair loss is definitely spinach. Because of its superior nutrient content, this is one of the best leafy green choices you can make when it comes to hair loss. Some of the other foods that will help you to have healthy hair are: seeds loaded with omega-3 fatty acids, guava, bok choy, sweet potatoes, apples, salmon, shiitake mushrooms, and eggs.

Finding the time to consume these foods during the day can be difficult and that's why it can be very useful to juice many of the fruits and vegetables that are beneficial to your hair. It only takes a couple of minutes to prepare most juices and the health benefits are absolutely amazing.

Having this in mind, I have created a collection of powerful superfood juices that are based on carefully chosen ingredients to improve your entire health and prevent hair loss. These juices will strengthen your immune system and give you shiny and beautiful hair.

53 HAIR LOSS JUICE RECIPE SOLUTIONS: JUICE YOUR WAY TO HEALTHIER AND STRONGER HAIR USING NATURES INGREDIENTS

1.   Spinach Carrot Juice

Ingredients:

1 cup of fresh spinach, torn

1 large carrot, chopped

1 cup of sweet potatoes, cubed

1 large banana, sliced

1 whole lime, peeled

1 small ginger knob, peeled

Preparation:

Wash the spinach thoroughly under cold running water. Slightly drain and torn with hands. Set aside.

Wash and peel the carrot. Cut into thin slices and set aside.

Peel the sweet potato and cut into small cubes. Fill the measuring cup and reserve the rest for later. Set aside.

Peel the banana and chop into chunks. Set aside.

Peel the lime and cut lengthwise in half. Set aside.

Peel the ginger knob and set aside.

Now, combine spinach, carrots, sweet potatoes, banana, lime, and ginger in a juicer and process until juiced. Transfer to a serving glass and refrigerate for 15 minutes before serving.

Enjoy!

Nutrition information per serving: Kcal: 270, Protein: 10.5g, Carbs: 77.1g, Fats: 1.6g

2. Orange Celery Juice

Ingredients:

1 small orange, wedged

2 medium-sized celery stalk

1 small apple, cored

1 large strawberry, chopped

Preparation:

Peel the orange and divide into wedges. Set aside.

Wash the celery and cut into bite-sized pieces. Set aside.

Wash the apple and cut in half. Remove the core and cut into bite-sized pieces. Set aside.

Wash the strawberry and cut in half. Set aside.

Now, combine orange, celery, apple, and strawberry in a juicer and process until well juiced. Transfer to a serving glass and add some crushed ice.

Serve immediately.

Nutrition information per serving: Kcal: 116, Protein: 2.2g, Carbs: 34.6g, Fats: 0.6g

3. Cauliflower Carrot Juice

Ingredients:

2 cauliflower flowerets, chopped

2 small carrots, chopped

1 cup of blackberries

1 cup of cucumber, sliced

1 cup of fresh kale, torn

Preparation:

Wash the cauliflower thoroughly and chop into small pieces. Set aside.

Wash and peel the carrots. Cut into thin slices and set aside.

Place the blackberries in a colander and rinse under cold running water. Slightly drain and set aside.

Wash the cucumber and cut into thin slices. Fill the measuring cup and reserve the rest for later.

Rinse the kale thoroughly and slightly drain. Torn with hands and set aside.

Now, combine cauliflower, carrots, blackberries, cucumber, and kale in a juicer and process until juiced.

Transfer to a serving glass and serve cold.

Nutrition information per serving: Kcal: 94, Protein: 6.4g, Carbs: 32.5g, Fats: 1.7g

4.   Orange Lemon Juice

Ingredients:

1 large orange, wedged

2 whole lemons, peeled

1 whole lime, peeled

1 small ginger slice, peeled

1 oz of water

Preparation:

Peel the orange and divide into wedges. Cut each wedge in half and set aside.

Peel the lemons and lime. Cut each fruit lengthwise in half and set aside.

Peel the ginger slice and set aside.

Now, combine orange, lemons, lime, and ginger in a juicer and process until well juiced. Add some ice and water to the juicer and reblend.

Transfer to a serving glass and garnish with some lemon or lime slices before serving.

Enjoy!

Nutrition information per serving: Kcal: 102, Protein: 3.3g, Carbs: 36.5g, Fats: 0.6g

5.   Avocado Broccoli Juice

Ingredients:

1 cup of avocado, cubed

1 cup of broccoli, chopped

1 small zucchini, cubed

1 cup of pomegranate seeds

Preparation:

Peel the avocado cut lengthwise in half. Remove the pit and cut into small cubes. Fill the measuring cup and reserve the rest for later. Set aside.

Wash the broccoli and cut into small pieces. Set aside.

Wash and peel the zucchini. Cut into small cubes and set aside.

Cut the top of the pomegranate fruit using a sharp paring knife. Slice down to each of the white membranes inside of the fruit. Pop the seeds into a measuring cup and set aside.

Now, combine avocado, broccoli, zucchini, and pomegranate seeds in a juicer and process until juiced.

Transfer to a serving glass and add some ice before serving. Garnish with some fresh mint, if you like. However, it's optional.

Enjoy!

Nutrition information per serving: Kcal: 294, Protein: 8.5g, Carbs: 38.7g, Fats: 23.7g

6. Mango Mint Juice

Ingredients:

1 cup of mango, cubed

1 cup of fresh mint, torn

1 large banana, sliced

1 whole grapefruit, wedged

1 oz of coconut water

Preparation:

Peel the mango and cut into small cubes. Fill the measuring cup and reserve the rest for later.

Wash the mint thoroughly and torn with hands. Set aside.

Peel the banana and cut into thin slices. Set aside.

Peel the grapefruit and divide into wedges. Cut each wedge in half and set aside.

Now, combine mango, mint, banana, and grapefruit in a juicer and process until juiced. Transfer to a serving glass and stir in the coconut water. Add some ice and serve immediately.

Enjoy!

Nutrition information per serving: Kcal: 293, Protein: 5.6g, Carbs: 85.7g, Fats: 1.6g

7.   Coriander Spinach Juice

Ingredients:

1 cup of fresh coriander, chopped

1 cup of fresh spinach, torn

1 cup of Romaine lettuce, shredded

1 whole cucumber, sliced

¼ tsp of salt

Preparation:

Combine coriander, spinach, and lettuce in a large colander. Wash thoroughly under cold running water and slightly drain. Roughly chop all and set aside.

Wash the cucumber and cut into thin slices. Set aside.

Now, combine coriander, spinach, lettuce, and cucumber in a juicer and process until well juiced.

Transfer to a serving glass and stir in the salt.

Serve immediately.

Nutrition information per serving: Kcal: 85, Protein: 10.3g, Carbs: 23.9g, Fats: 1.8g

8.   Carrot Lime Juice

Ingredients:

2 medium-sized carrots, sliced

1 whole lime, peeled

1 cup of cucumber, sliced

1 medium-sized orange, wedged

1 tbsp of honey

Preparation:

Wash and peel the carrots. Cut into thin slices and set aside.

Peel the lime and cut lengthwise in half. Set aside.

Wash the cucumber and cut into thin slices. Fill the measuring cup and reserve the rest for later.

Peel the orange and divide into wedges. Cut each wedge in half and set aside.

Now, combine carrots, lime, cucumber, and orange in a juicer and process until juiced. Transfer to a serving glass and stir in the honey.

Add some ice before serving.

Enjoy!

Nutrition information per serving: Kcal: 163, Protein: 2.9g, Carbs: 32.6g, Fats: 0.6g

9.   Beet Grapefruit Juice

Ingredients:

1 cup of beets, trimmed and sliced

1 whole grapefruit, peeled

1 cup of avocado, cubed

½ cup of green grapes

Preparation:

Wash the beets thoroughly and trim off the green parts, Cut into thin slices and fill the measuring cup. Reserve the rest in the refrigerator.

Peel the grapefruit and divide into wedges. Cut each wedge in half and set aside.

Peel the avocado and cut lengthwise in half. Cut into small cubes and fill the measuring cup. Reserve the rest for later.

Wash the grapes and fill the measuring cup. Set aside.

now, combine beets, grapefruit, avocado, and grapes in a juicer. Add few ice cubes and process until juiced.

Transfer to a serving glass and serve immediately.

Nutrition information per serving: Kcal: 350, Protein: 7.3g, Carbs: 56.1g, Fats: 22.6g

10.   Tomato Parsley Juice

Ingredients:

5 cherry tomatoes, halved

1 cup of fresh parsley, finely chopped

1 cup of cucumber, sliced

1 large red bell pepper, chopped

1 whole lemon, peeled

1 tsp of fresh rosemary, finely chopped

Preparation:

Wash the cherry tomatoes and place in a bowl. Cut each tomato in half and make sure to reserve the tomato juice.

Wash the parsley thoroughly under cold running water and slightly drain. Roughly chop it and set aside.

Wash the cucumber and cut into thin slices. Fill the measuring cup and reserve the rest for later.

Wash the bell pepper and cut in half. Remove the seeds and chop into small pieces. Set aside.

Peel the lemon and cut lengthwise in half. Set aside.

Now, combine cherry tomatoes, parsley, cucumber, bell pepper, lemon, and rosemary in a juicer and process until well juiced. Transfer to a serving glass and refrigerate for 10 minutes before serving.

Nutrition information per serving: Kcal: 79, Protein: 5.1g, Carbs: 24.9g, Fats: 1.3g

11. Mango Banana Juice

Ingredients:

1 cup of mango, chunked

1 medium-sized banana, sliced

1 small apple, cored

1 cup of fresh mint, torn

1 small ginger knob, peeled

1 tbsp of liquid honey

Preparation:

Peel the mango and cut into small chunks. Fill the measuring cup and reserve the rest for later. Set aside.

Peel the banana and cut into thin slices. Set aside.

Wash the apple and cut in half. Remove the core and cut into bite-sized pieces. Set aside.

Place the mint in a large colander. Rinse well under cold running water and slightly drain. Torn with hands and set aside.

Peel the ginger knob and set aside.

Now, combine mango, banana, apple, mint, and ginger in a juicer and process until juiced. Transfer to a serving glass and stir in the honey.

Add few ice cubes and serve immediately.

Nutrition information per serving: Kcal: 325, Protein: 4.3g, Carbs: 76.1g, Fats: 1.6g

12.   Broccoli Cabbage Juice

Ingredients:

1 cup of broccoli, chopped

1 cup of purple cabbage, torn

1 whole beet, chopped

1 cup of Swiss chard, torn

1 cup of cucumber, sliced

¼ tsp of turmeric, ground

Preparation:

Wash the broccoli and trim off the outer layers. Chop it into small pieces and set aside.

Combine purple cabbage and Swiss chard in a large colander. Wash thoroughly under cold running water and slightly drain. Torn with hands and set aside.

Wash the beets and trim off the green parts. Cut into bite-sized pieces and set aside.

Wash the cucumber and cut into thin slices. Fill the measuring cup and reserve the rest for later. Set aside.

Now, combine broccoli, purple cabbage, beet, Swiss chard, and cucumber in a juicer and process until juiced.

Transfer to a serving glass and stir in the turmeric. Refrigerate for 15 minutes and serve.

Enjoy!

Nutrition information per serving: Kcal: 79, Protein: 6.2g, Carbs: 23.7g, Fats: 0.8g

13.   Artichoke Orange Juice

Ingredients:

1 medium-sized artichoke, chopped

1 small orange, peeled

1 whole lemon, peeled

1 whole lime, peeled

1 tbsp of liquid honey

1 oz of water

Preparation:

Trim off the outer layers of the artichoke using a sharp paring knife. Cut into bite-sized pieces and set aside.

Peel the orange and divide into wedges. Cut each wedge in half and set aside.

Peel the lemon and lime. Cut each fruit lengthwise in half and set aside.

Now, combine artichoke, orange, lemon, and lime in a juicer. Process until well juiced. Transfer to a serving glass and stir in the honey and water.

Refrigerate for 10 minutes before serving.

Nutrition information per serving: Kcal: 149, Protein: 5.9g, Carbs: 33.8g, Fats: 0.5g

14. Honeydew Melon Juice

Ingredients:

1 medium-sized slice of honeydew melon

1 medium-sized carrot, sliced

1 medium-sized peach, chopped

1 small green apple, cored

Preparation:

Cut melon lengthwise in half. Scoop out the seeds and then wash the melon. Cut one wedge and peel it. Cut into bite-sized pieces and set aside.

Wash and peel the carrot. Cut into thin slices and set aside.

Wash the peach and cut in half. Remove the pit and cut small pieces. Set aside.

Wash the apple and cut in half. Remove the core and cut into bite-sized pieces. Set aside.

Now, combine melon, carrot, peach, and apple in a juicer and process until juiced. Transfer to a serving glass and refrigerate for 10 minutes before serving.

Nutrition information per serving: Kcal: 176, Protein: 3.2g, Carbs: 51.1g, Fats: 1g

15. Blueberry Lemon Juice

Ingredients:

1 cup of blueberries

1 whole lemon, peeled

1 large banana, sliced

1 large pear, chopped

2 oz of coconut water

Preparation:

Place the blueberries in a colander and rinse under cold water. Slightly drain and set aside.

Peel the lemon and cut lengthwise in half. Set aside.

Peel the banana and cut into thin slices. Set aside.

Wash the pear and cut in half. Remove the core and cut into bite-sized pieces. Set aside.

Now, combine blueberries, lemon, banana, and pear in a juicer and process until juiced. Transfer to a serving glass and stir in the coconut water. Add some ice and serve immediately.

Enjoy!

Nutrition information per serving: Kcal: 291, Protein: 4.1g, Carbs: 92.3g, Fats: 1.4g

16. Cherry Cantaloupe Juice

Ingredients:

1 cup of cherries, pitted

1 small cantaloupe wedge

1 whole lemon, peeled

1 cup of pineapple chunks

Preparation:

Wash the cherries and remove the green stems, if any. Cut each cherry in half and fill the measuring cup. Set aside.

Cut the cantaloupe in half. Scrape out the seeds and cut one thin slice. Wrap the rest in a plastic foil and refrigerate for later.

Peel the lemon and cut lengthwise in half. Set aside.

Using a sharp paring knife, cut the top of the pineapple. Gently remove all hard skin and slice it into thin slices. Fill the measuring cup and reserve the rest for later.

Now, combine cherries, cantaloupe, lemon, and pineapple in a juicer. Process until well juiced. Transfer to a serving glass and refrigerate for 10 minutes before serving. Enjoy!

Nutrition information per serving: Kcal: 176, Protein: 3.4g, Carbs: 53.6g, Fats: 0.7g

17.   Pepper Greens Juice

Ingredients:

1 large red bell pepper, chopped

1 cup of collard greens, chopped

1 cup of fennel, chopped

1 large radish, chopped

1 whole lemon, peeled

1 small ginger knob, peeled

1 oz of water

Preparation:

Wash the bell pepper and cut in half. Remove the seeds and chop into small pieces. Set aside.

Wash the collard greens and chop into small pieces. Set aside.

Trim off the outer wilted layers of the fennel. Roughly chop it and fill the measuring cup. Reserve the rest for later.

Wash the radish and trim off the green ends. Slightly peel it and chop into small pieces. Set aside.

Peel the lemon and cut lengthwise in half. Set aside.

Peel the ginger knob and roughly chop it. Set aside.

Now, combine bell pepper, collard greens, fennel, radish, lemon, and ginger in a juicer. Process until juiced.

Transfer to a serving glass and stir in the water. Refrigerate for 10 minutes before serving.

Nutrition information per serving: Kcal: 76, Protein: 4.6g, Carbs: 24.9g, Fats: 1.1g

18. Cauliflower Kale Juice

Ingredients:

1 cup of cauliflower, chopped

1 cup of fresh kale, chopped

1 whole lime, peeled

1 cup of cucumber, sliced

¼ tsp of salt

Preparation:

Trim off the outer layer of the cauliflower. Cut into bite-sized pieces and wash it. Fill the measuring cup and sprinkle with some salt. Set aside.

Wash the kale thoroughly under cold running water and slightly drain. Chop into small pieces and set aside.

Peel the lime and cut lengthwise in half. Set aside.

Wash the cucumber and cut into thin slices. Fill the measuring cup and reserve the rest for some other juice. Set aside.

Now, combine cauliflower, kale, lime, and cucumber in a juicer. Process until well juiced. Transfer to a serving glass and refrigerate before serving.

Enjoy!

Nutrition information per serving: Kcal: 87, Protein: 11.4g, Carbs: 24.4g, Fats: 1.8g

19.   Avocado Carrot Juice

Ingredients:

1 cup of avocado, chunked

1 large carrot, sliced

1 small red apple, cored

½ cup of green grapes

1 whole kiwi, peeled

¼ tsp of ginger, ground

Preparation:

Peel the avocado and cut in half. Remove the pit and cut into small chunks. Fill the measuring cup and reserve the rest for later.

Wash and peel the carrot. Cut into thin slices and set aside.

Wash the apple and cut in half. Remove the core and cut into bite-sized pieces. Set aside.

Peel the kiwi and cut lengthwise in half. Set aside.

now, combine avocado, carrot, apple, grapes, and kiwi in a juicer and process until juiced. Transfer to a serving glass and stir in the ginger.

Add some crushed ice and serve immediately.

Nutrition information per serving: Kcal: 355, Protein: 5.1g, Carbs: 56.1g, Fats: 22.9g

20.   Grapefruit Cherry Juice

Ingredients:

1 whole grapefruit, peeled

1 cup of cherries, pitted

1 medium-sized banana, sliced

1 cup of fresh mint, torn

2 tbsp of coconut water

Preparation:

Peel the grapefruit and divide into wedges. Cut each wedge in half and set aside.

Wash the cherries and remove the stems, if any. Cut each cherry in half and remove the pits. Fill the measuring cup and set aside.

Peel the banana and cut into thin slices. Set aside.

Wash the mint thoroughly under cold running water and slightly drain. Torn with hands and set aside.

Now, combine grapefruit, cherries, banana, and mint in a juicer and process until juiced. Transfer to a serving glass and stir in the coconut water.

Add some crushed ice and serve immediately.

Nutrition information per serving: Kcal: 274, Protein: 5.8g, Carbs: 81.5g, Fats: 1.3g

21.   Apple Kiwi Juice

Ingredients:

1 small apple, cored

1 whole kiwi, peeled

 1 small peach, pitted

½ cup of fresh spinach, torn

Preparation:

Wash the apple and cut in half. Remove the core and cut into bite-sized pieces. Set aside.

Peel the kiwi and cut lengthwise in half. Set aside.

Wash the peach and cut in half. Remove the pit and cut into bite-sized pieces. Set aside.

Rinse the spinach under cold running water and slightly drain. Torn with hands and set aside.

Now, combine apple, kiwi, peach, and spinach in a juicer and process until juiced. Transfer to a serving glass and add some ice.

Serve immediately.

Nutrition information per serving: Kcal: 165, Protein: 6.9g, Carbs: 47.6g, Fats: 1.5g

22.   Parsnip Beet Juice

Ingredients:

1 cup of parsnip, sliced

1 cup of beets, sliced

1 cup of sweet potatoes, chunked

1 cup of mustard greens, torn

1 cup of watercress, torn

Preparation:

Wash and peel the parsnips. Remove the green parts and cut into thin slices. Fill the measuring cup and reserve the rest for later.

Wash the beets and trim off the green ends. Slightly peel and cut into thin slices. Fill the measuring cup and set aside.

Peel the potato and cut into small chunks. Fill the measuring cup and reserve the rest for later.

Combine mustard greens and watercress in a colander. Wash thoroughly under cold running water and slightly drain. Torn with hands and set aside.

Now, combine parsnips, beets, sweet potatoes, mustard greens, and watercress in a juicer and process until juiced.

Transfer to a serving glass and add some salt if you like. However, it is optional.

Nutrition information per serving: Kcal: 226, Protein: 8.3g, Carbs: 66.7g, Fats: 0.9g

23.   Watermelon Blackberry Juice

Ingredients:

1 cup of watermelon, cubed

1 cup of blackberries

1 medium-sized orange, peeled

1 tbsp of liquid honey

¼ tsp of cinnamon, ground

Preparation:

Cut the watermelon in half. Cut one large wedge and wrap the rest in a plastic foil and refrigerate. Peel the slice and cut into small cubes. Remove the pits and fill the measuring cup. Set aside.

Wash the blackberries thoroughly under cold water and slightly drain. Set aside.

Peel the orange and divide into wedges. Cut each wedge in half and set aside.

Now, combine watermelon, blackberries, and orange in a juicer and process until juiced. Transfer to a serving glass and stir in the honey and cinnamon.

Refrigerate for 10 minutes before serving.

Enjoy!

Nutrition information per serving: Kcal: 186, Protein: 4.2g, Carbs: 40.7g, Fats: 1.1g

24. Cranberry Raspberry Juice

Ingredients:

1 cup of cranberries

1 cup of raspberries

1 cup of fresh mint, torn

1 whole lemon, peeled

1 small apple, cored

Preparation:

Combine cranberries and raspberries in a large colander. Wash thoroughly under cold running water and slightly drain. Set aside.

Wash the mint and torn with hands. Set aside.

Peel the lemon and cut lengthwise in half. Set aside.

Wash the apple and cut in half. Remove the core and cut into bite-sized pieces.

Now, combine cranberries, raspberries, mint, lemon, and apple in a juicer and process until juiced. Transfer to a serving glass and add some ice before serving.

Enjoy!

Nutrition information per serving: Kcal: 143, Protein: 3.8g, Carbs: 53.5g, Fats: 1.5g

25. Strawberry Banana Juice

Ingredients:

1 cup of strawberries, chopped

1 medium-sized banana, sliced

1 whole grapefruit, wedged

1 small Granny Smith's apple, cored

1 tbsp of coconut water

Preparation:

Wash the strawberries and remove the stems. Cut into bite-sized pieces and fill the measuring cup. Reserve the rest for later.

Peel the banana and cut into thin slices. Set aside.

Peel the grapefruit and divide into wedges. Cut each wedge in half and set aside.

Wash the apple and cut lengthwise in half. Remove the core and cut into bite-sized pieces. Set aside.

Now, combine strawberries, banana, grapefruit, and apple in a juicer and process until well juiced. Transfer to a serving glass and stir in the coconut water.

Add few ice cubes and serve immediately.

Nutrition information per serving: Kcal: 268, Protein: 4.4g, Carbs: 79.6g, Fats: 1.2g

26.   Guava Mango Juice

Ingredients:

1 whole guava, peeled

1 medium-sized orange, peeled

1 large carrot, sliced

1 whole lemon, peeled

1 tbsp of liquid honey

Preparation:

Peel the guava with a sharp paring knife. Cut into small chunks and set aside.

Peel the orange and divide into wedges. Cut each wedge in half and set aside.

Wash and peel the carrot. Cut into thin slices and set aside.

Peel the lemon and cut lengthwise in half. Set aside.

Now, combine guava, orange, carrot, and lemon in a juicer and process until juiced. Transfer to a serving glass and stir in the honey. Add some ice and serve immediately.

Nutrition information per serving: Kcal: 168, Protein: 3.9g, Carbs: 35.6g, Fats: 1.1g

27. Pineapple Cherry Juice

Ingredients:

1 cup of pineapple, chunked

1 cup of cherries, pitted

1 medium-sized carrot, sliced

¼ tsp of ginger, ground

1 tbsp of coconut water

Preparation:

Using a sharp paring knife, cut the top of the pineapple. Gently remove all hard skin and slice it into thin slices. Fill the measuring cup and reserve the rest for later.

Wash the cherries and cut each in half. Remove the pits and fill the measuring cup. Reserve the rest in the refrigerator.

Wash and peel the carrot. Cut into thin slices and set aside.

Now, combine pineapple, cherries, and carrot in a juicer and process until well juiced. Transfer to a serving glass and stir in the ginger and coconut water. Garnish with some fresh mint and serve immediately.

Nutrition information per serving: Kcal: 175, Protein: 3.1g, Carbs: 52.1g, Fats: 0.6g

28. Zucchini Asparagus Juice

Ingredients:

1 small zucchini, chopped

2 medium-sized asparagus spears

1 cup of celery, chopped

1 cup of fresh basil, torn

1 whole lime, peeled

Preparation:

Wash the zucchini and cut into bite-sized pieces. Set aside.

Wash the asparagus and trim off the woody ends. Cut into small pieces and set aside.

Wash the celery and remove the white parts. Cut the green parts into small pieces. Set aside.

Rinse the basil under cold running water using a colander. Slightly drain and torn with hands. Set aside.

Peel the lime and cut lengthwise in half. Set aside.

Now, combine zucchini, asparagus, celery, basil, and lime in a juicer and process until juiced. Transfer to a serving glass and add some ice before serving.

Enjoy!

Nutrition information per serving: Kcal: 43, Protein: 3.7g, Carbs: 12.3g, Fats: 0.7g

29.   Mango Pear Juice

Ingredients:

1 cup of mango, chunked

1 medium-sized pear, chopped

1 cup of pomegranate seeds

1 cup of Romaine lettuce, shredded

1 tbsp of liquid honey

Preparation:

Peel the mango and cut into small chunks. Fill the measuring cup and reserve the rest in the refrigerator. Set aside.

Wash the pear and cut into small pieces. Set aside.

Cut the top of the pomegranate fruit using a sharp paring knife. Slice down to each of the white membranes inside of the fruit. Pop the seeds into a measuring cup and set aside.

Wash the lettuce thoroughly under cold running water and shred it. Fill the measuring cup and reserve the rest for later.

Now, combine mango, pear, pomegranate, and lettuce in a juicer and process until well juiced. Transfer to a serving glass and stir in the honey. Add some ice and serve immediately.

Nutrition information per serving: Kcal: 230, Protein: 4.1g, Carbs: 69.6g, Fats: 2.1g

30.   Plum Kiwi Juice

Ingredients:

2 large plums, pitted

1 whole kiwi, peeled

1 cup of cantaloupe, chunked

1 cup of red leaf lettuce, shredded

1 tbsp of liquid honey

Preparation:

Wash the plums and cut in half. Remove the pits and cut into bite-sized pieces. Set aside.

Peel the kiwi and cut lengthwise in half. Set aside.

Cut the cantaloupe in half. Scoop out the seeds and flesh. Cut two wedges and peel them. Chop into chunks and set aside. Reserve the rest of the cantaloupe in a refrigerator.

Wash the lettuce thoroughly and shred it. Fill the measuring cup and reserve the rest for later.

Now, combine plums, kiwi, cantaloupe, and lettuce in a juicer and process until juiced. Transfer to a serving glass and stir in the honey.

Add some ice and serve immediately.

Nutrition information per serving: Kcal: 136, Protein: 3.4g, Carbs: 38.6g, Fats: 1.1g

31.   Basil Tomato Juice

Ingredients:

1 cup of fresh basil, torn

5 cherry tomatoes, halved

1 cup of fresh parsley, torn

1 cup of fresh spinach, chopped

1 cup of mustard greens, torn

¼ tsp of salt

Preparation:

Combine basil, parsley, and mustard greens in a colander.Rinse well under cold running water and slightly drain. Torn with hands and set aside.

Wash the spinach leaves and chop into small pieces. Fill the measuring cup and reserve the rest for later. Set aside.

Wash the cherry tomatoes and remove the stems. Place in a small bowl and cut in half. Make sure to reserve the juice while cutting. Set aside.

Now, combine basil, parsley, mustard greens, spinach and tomatoes in a juicer and process until well juiced. Transfer to a serving glass and stir in the reserved tomato juice and salt.

Serve cold.

Nutrition information per serving: Kcal: 64, Protein: 10.9g, Carbs: 17.9g, Fats: 1.8g

32.   Orange Cantaloupe Juice

Ingredients:

1 large orange, peeled

1 medium-sized slice of cantaloupe

1 small ginger knob, peeled

1 cup of cucumber, sliced

1 tbsp of coconut water

Preparation:

Peel the orange and divide into wedges. Cut each wedge in half and set aside.

Cut the cantaloupe in half. Scoop out the seeds and cut the wedge. Peel it and cut into small pieces. Set aside.

Peel the ginger knob and cut in small pieces. Set aside.

Wash the cucumber and cut into thin slices. Fill the measuring cup and reserve the rest for later. Set aside.

Now, combine orange, cantaloupe, ginger, and cucumber in a juicer and process until juiced. Transfer to a serving glass and stir in the coconut water.

Refrigerate for 10 minutes before serving.

Nutrition information per serving: Kcal: 103, Protein: 2.7g, Carbs: 30.2g, Fats: 0.5g

33.   Pomegranate Watermelon Juice

Ingredients:

1 cup of pomegranate seeds

1 cup of watermelon, cubed

1 whole beet, sliced

1 cup of watercress, torn

Preparation:

Cut the top of the pomegranate fruit using a sharp paring knife. Slice down to each of the white membranes inside of the fruit. Pop the seeds into a measuring cup and set aside.

Cut the watermelon lengthwise in half. For one cup, you'll need about one large wedge. Cut and peel the wedge. Cut into bite-sized cubes and remove the seeds. Fill the measuring cup and set aside.

Wash and peel the beet. Remove the green parts and cut into small pieces. Set aside.

Wash the watercress thoroughly under cold running water and slightly drain. Torn with hands and set aside.

Now, combine pomegranate, watermelon, beets, and watercress in a juicer and process until well juiced.

Transfer to a serving glass and serve immediately.

Nutrition information per serving: Kcal: 131, Protein: 4.5g, Carbs: 36.1g, Fats: 1.4g

34.   Pepper Kale Juice

Ingredients:

2 medium-sized bell peppers, chopped

1 cup of fresh kale, chopped

1 large radish, trimmed

1 cup of avocado, cubed

1 cup of cucumber, sliced

Preparation:

Wash the bell peppers and cut lengthwise in half. Remove the seeds and cut into small pieces. Set aside.

Wash the kale under cold running water and slightly drain. Chop into small pieces and set aside.

Peel and wash the radish. Trim off the green parts and cut into small pieces. Set aside.

Peel the avocado and cut in half. Remove the pit and cut into small cubes. Fill the measuring cup and reserve the rest for later.

Wash the cucumber and cut into thin slices. Fill the measuring cup and reserve the rest for later. Set aside.

Now, combine bell peppers, kale, radish, avocado, and cucumber in a juicer and process until well juiced. Transfer to a serving glass and serve immediately.

Nutrition information per serving: Kcal: 131, Protein: 4.5g, Carbs: 36.1g, Fats: 1.4g

35. Apricot Cherry Juice

Ingredients:

1 cup of apricots, pitted

1 cup of cherries, pitted

1 small ginger slice, peeled

1 oz of coconut water

Preparation:

Wash the apricots and cut in half. Remove the pits and cut into small pieces. Fill the measuring cup and set aside.

Wash the cherries and remove the stems, if any. Cut each in half and remove the pits. Fill the measuring cup and set aside.

Peel the ginger slice and set aside.

Now, combine apricots, cherries, and ginger in a juicer and process until well juiced. Transfer to a serving glass and stir in the coconut water.

Refrigerate for 10 minutes before serving.

Enjoy!

Nutrition information per serving: Kcal: 149, Protein: 3.8g, Carbs: 40.8g, Fats: 0.9g

36.   Plum Cabbage Juice

Ingredients:

4 whole plums, chopped

1 cup of purple cabbage, shredded

1 cup of blueberries

1 whole lime, peeled

Preparation:

Wash the plums and cut each in half. Remove the pits and cut into bite-sized pieces. Set aside.

Wash the cabbage thoroughly and shred it. Fill the measuring cup and set aside. Reserve the rest for some other recipe.

Wash the blueberries and slightly drain. Set aside.

Peel the lime and cut lengthwise in half. Set aside.

Now, combine plums, cabbage, blueberries, and lime in a juicer and process until well juiced. Transfer to a serving glass and add some ice before serving.

Enjoy!

Nutrition information per serving: Kcal: 204, Protein: 4.4g, Carbs: 61.8g, Fats: 1.4g

37.   Papaya Orange Juice

Ingredients:

1 cup of papaya, peeled

1 large orange, wedged

1 whole lime, peeled

1 cup of fresh mint, torn

2 oz of coconut water

1 tbsp of liquid honey

Preparation:

Peel the papaya and cut in half. Scoop out the seeds and cut into small chunks. Set aside.

Peel the orange and divide into wedges. Cut each wedge in half and set aside.

Peel the lime and cut lengthwise in half. Set aside.

Wash the mint thoroughly under cold running water and slightly drain. Torn with hands and set aside.

Now, combine papaya, orange, lime, and mint in a juicer and process until well juiced. Transfer to a serving glass and stir in the coconut water.

Add some ice and serve immediately.

Enjoy!

Nutrition information per serving: Kcal: 200, Protein: 3.6g, Carbs: 44.7g, Fats: 0.9g

38.   Coriander Leek Juice

Ingredients:

1 cup of fresh coriander, chopped

2 whole leeks, chopped

1 cup of turnip greens, chopped

1 cup of sweet potatoes, cubed

1 cup of cucumber, sliced

1 whole lime, peeled

1 cup of spinach, chopped

Preparation:

In a large colander, combine coriander, turnip greens, and spinach. Wash thoroughly under cold running water. Chop all into small pieces and set aside.

Wash the leeks and cut into bite-sized pieces. Set aside.

Peel the sweet potato and cut into small cubes. Fill the measuring cup and reserve the rest for later. Set aside.

Wash the cucumber and cut into thin slices. fill the measuring cup and reserve the rest for later. Set aside.

Peel the lime and cut lengthwise in half. Set aside.

Now, combine coriander, turnip greens, spinach, leeks, sweet potatoes, and cucumber in a juicer. Process until well juiced.

Transfer to a serving glass and serve immediately.

Nutrition information per serving: Kcal: 264, Protein: 2.2g, Carbs: 72.8g, Fats: 13.9g

39.   Broccoli Zucchini Juice

Ingredients:

1 cup of broccoli, chopped

1 small zucchini, chopped

1 cup of green peas

1 cup of Brussels sprouts

1 cup of cucumber, sliced

1 small ginger slice, peeled

Preparation:

Wash the broccoli and trim off the outer layers. Cut into small pieces and set aside.

Peel the zucchini and cut into bite-sized pieces. Set aside.

Wash the Brussels sprouts and trim off the outer wilted leaves. Cut in half and set aside.

Wash the cucumber and cut into thin slices. Fill the measuring cup and reserve the rest for later. Set aside.

Now, combine broccoli, zucchini, Brussels sprouts, and cucumber in a juicer and process until well juiced. Transfer to a serving glass and serve immediately.

Nutrition information per serving: Kcal: 160, Protein: 15.3g, Carbs: 41.5g, Fats: 1.6g

40.   Avocado Plum Juice

Ingredients:

1 cup of avocado, cubed

2 whole plums, chopped

1 medium-sized apple, cored

1 whole lemon, peeled

¼ tsp of cinnamon, ground

1 tbsp of coconut water

Preparation:

Peel the avocado and cut in half. Remove the pit and cut into small cubes. Fill the measuring cup and reserve the rest for later.

Wash the plums and cut lengthwise in half. Remove the pits and cut into bite-sized pieces. Set aside.

Wash the apple and cut in half. Remove the pit and cut into small pieces. Set aside.

Peel the lemon and cut into half. Set aside.

Now, combine avocado, plums, apple, and lemon in a juicer and process until juiced. Transfer to a serving glass and stir in the cinnamon and coconut water.

Refrigerate for 15 minutes before serving.

Enjoy!

Nutrition information per serving: Kcal: 341, Protein: 5.3g, Carbs: 56.1g, Fats: 22.8g

41.   Pumpkin Apple Juice

Ingredients:

1 cup of pumpkin, cubed

1 small Granny Smith's apple, cored

1 medium-sized carrot, sliced

1 cup of cucumber, sliced

¼ tsp of cinnamon, ground

¼ tsp of ginger, ground

Preparation:

Cut the pumpkin in half and scoop out the seeds. Wash it and cut one large wedge. Peel it and cut into small cubes. Fill the measuring cup and reserve the rest in the refrigerator.

Wash the apple and cut lengthwise in half. Remove the core and cut into small pieces. Set aside.

Wash and peel the carrot. Cut into thin slices and set aside.

Wash the cucumber and cut into thin slices. Fill the measuring cup and reserve the rest for later.

Now, combine pumpkin, apple, carrot, and cucumber in a juicer and process until juiced. Transfer to a serving glass and stir in the cinnamon and ginger.

Refrigerate for 10 minutes before serving.

Nutritional information per serving: Kcal: 121, Protein: 2.7g, Carbs: 34.8g, Fats: 0.6g

42.   Peach Lime Juice

Ingredients:

2 large peaches, pitted

1 whole lime, peeled

1 cup of apricots, sliced

1 large banana, peeled

Preparation:

Wash the peaches and cut in half. Remove the pits and cut each half into bite-sized pieces. Set aside.

Peel the lime and roughly chop it. Make sure to reserve lime juice while cutting.

Wash the apricots and cut in half. Remove the pits and cut into small pieces. Fill the measuring cup and set aside.

Peel the banana and cut into small chunks. Set aside.

Now, combine peaches, lime, apricots, and banana in a juicer and process until juiced. Transfer to a serving glass and add some crushed ice before serving.

Enjoy!

Nutritional information per serving: Kcal: 299, Protein: 7.2g, Carbs: 86.5g, Fats: 2g

43.   Artichoke Spinach Juice

Ingredients:

1 medium-sized artichoke, chopped

1 cup of fresh spinach, chopped

1 cup of green beans, chopped

1 small green bell pepper, sliced

1 small ginger knob, peeled and sliced

Preparation:

Trim off the outer leaves of the artichoke using a sharp paring knife. Wash it and cut into bite-sized pieces. Set aside.

Using a colander, rinse the spinach thoroughly under cold running water. Chop into small pieces and set aside.

Place the beans in a deep pot. Add 1 cup of water and bring it to a boil. Cook for 5 minutes and remove from the heat. Set aside to cool completely.

Wash the bell pepper and cut in half. Remove the seeds and stem. Cut into small rings and set aside.

Peel the ginger knob and chop it into small pieces. Set aside.

Now, combine artichoke, spinach, green beans, bell pepper, and ginger in a juicer and process until juiced. Transfer to a serving glass and refrigerate for 10 minutes before serving.

Nutritional information per serving: Kcal: 95, Protein: 11.9g, Carbs: 29.4g, Fats: 1.3g

44. Orange Pear Juice

Ingredients:

1 medium-sized orange, peeled

1 medium-sized pear, chopped

1 whole plum, pitted

1 whole lemon, peeled

1 oz of water

Preparation:

Peel the orange and divide into wedges. Cut each wedge in half and set aside.

Wash the pear and cut in half. Remove the core and chop into small pieces. Set aside.

Wash the plum and cut in half. Remove the pit and cut in small pieces.

Peel the lemon and cut into quarters. Set aside.

Now, combine orange, pear, plum, and lemon in a juicer and process until juiced. Transfer to a serving glass and stir in the water.

You can add a pinch of minced mint for some extra smooth flavor, but it's optional.

Add some crushed ice and serve immediately.

Nutritional information per serving: Kcal: 166, Protein: 2.9g, Carbs: 55.4g, Fats: 0.8g

45. Carrot Grapefruit Juice

Ingredients:

2 medium-sized carrots, sliced

1 whole grapefruit, wedged

1 cup of Romaine lettuce, shredded

1 cup of fresh mint, chopped

1 whole lime, peeled

Preparation:

Wash and peel the carrots. Cut into thin slices and set aside.

Peel the grapefruit and divide into wedges. Cut each wedge in half and set aside.

Wash the lettuce thoroughly under cold running water. Shred it and fill the measuring cup. Reserve the rest for later.

Wash the mint and then place it in a medium bowl. Add one cup of hot water and let it soak for 10 minutes. Slightly drain and set aside.

Peel the lime and cut lengthwise in half. Set aside.

Now, combine carrots, grapefruit, lettuce, mint, and lime in a juicer and process until juiced. Transfer to a serving glass and add some crushed ice before serving.

Enjoy!

Nutritional information per serving: Kcal: 147, Protein: 4.7g, Carbs: 46.8g, Fats: 1.1g

46. Swiss Chard Juice

Ingredients:

2 cups of Swiss chard, chopped

1 cup of fresh kale, chopped

1 cup of collard greens, chopped

1 whole lemon, peeled

1 cup of cucumber, sliced

¼ tsp of ginger, ground

Preparation:

Combine Swiss chard, kale, and collard greens in a large colander. Wash thoroughly under cold running water. Slightly drain and roughly chop all. Set aside.

Peel the lemon and cut lengthwise in half. Set aside.

Wash the cucumber and cut into thin slices. Fill the measuring cup and reserve the rest in the refrigerator. Set aside.

Now, combine Swiss chard, kale, collard greens, lemon, and cucumber in a juicer. Process until juiced.

Transfer to a serving glass and stir in the ginger.

Serve cold.

Nutritional information per serving: Kcal: 57, Protein: 6.3g, Carbs: 17.8g, Fats: 1.2g

47. Broccoli Brussels Sprout Juice

Ingredients:

1 cup of broccoli, chopped

1 cup of Brussels sprouts, halved

1 cup of cucumber, sliced

1 whole lime, peeled

¼ tsp of ginger, ground

Preparation:

Wash the broccoli and trim off the outer layers. Cut into small pieces and fill the measuring cup. Set aside.

Wash the Brussels sprouts and trim off the outer leaves. Cut each sprout in half and fill the measuring cup. Reserve the rest for in the refrigerator.

Wash the cucumber and cut into thin slices. Fill the measuring cup and reserve the rest for later. Set aside.

Peel the lime and cut lengthwise in half.

Now, combine broccoli, Brussels sprouts, cucumber, and lime in a juicer and process until juiced. Transfer to a serving glass and stir in the ginger.

Add few ice cubes and serve immediately.

Nutritional information per serving: Kcal: 63, Protein: 6.1g, Carbs: 19.5g, Fats: 1.2g

48. Blackberry Avocado Juice

Ingredients:

2 cups of blackberries

1 cup of avocado, cubed

1 medium-sized apple, cored

¼ tsp of ginger, ground

Preparation:

Place the blackberries in a colander and wash thoroughly under cold running water. Slightly drain and set aside.

Peel the avocado and cut lengthwise in half. Remove the pit and cut into small cubes. Fill the measuring cup and reserve the rest in the refrigerator.

Wash the apple and cut in half. Remove the core and cut into bite-sized pieces. Set aside.

Now, combine blackberries, avocado, and apple in a juicer and process until juiced. Transfer to a serving glass and stir in the ginger.

Add some ice and serve immediately.

Nutritional information per serving: Kcal: 342, Protein: 7.7g, Carbs: 63.2g, Fats: 23.7g

49. Raspberry Pear Juice

Ingredients:

1 cup of raspberries

1 large pear, chopped

1 whole lemon, peeled

1 small green apple, cored

Preparation:

Wash the raspberries thoroughly using a colander. Slightly drain and set aside.

Wash the pear and cut in half. Remove the core and cut into bite-sized pieces. Set aside.

Peel the lemon and cut lengthwise in half. Set aside.

Wash the apple and cut in half. Remove the core and cut into small pieces. Set aside.

Now, combine raspberries, pear, lemon, and apple in a juicer and process until juiced. Transfer to a serving glass and add some ice before serving.

Enjoy!

Nutritional information per serving: Kcal: 214, Protein: 3.6g, Carbs: 74.7g, Fats: 1.6g

50. Coco Squash Juice

Ingredients:

1 cup of crookneck squash, sliced

1 medium-sized pear, chopped

1 cup of cucumber, sliced

1 whole lime, peeled

1 oz of coconut water

Preparation:

Peel the crookneck squash and scrape out the seeds with a spoon. Cut into small cubes and fill the measuring cup. Reserve the rest of the squash for some other recipe. Wrap in a plastic foil and refrigerate.

Wash the pear and cut in half. Remove the core and chop into small pieces. Set aside.

Wash the cucumber and cut into thin slices. Fill the measuring cup and reserve the rest in the refrigerator. Set aside.

Peel the lime and cut lengthwise in half. Set aside.

Now, combine squash, pear, cucumber, and lime in a juicer. Process until juiced. Transfer to a serving glass and stir in the coconut water.

Add some ice and serve immediately.

Nutritional information per serving: Kcal: 120, Protein: 2.4g, Carbs: 37.6g, Fats: 0.7g

51.   Kiwi Papaya Juice

Ingredients:

4 whole kiwis, peeled

2 small papaya, chopped

1 tbsp of fresh basil, roughly chopped

1 large banana, peeled

1 cup of cucumber, sliced

Preparation:

Peel the kiwis and cut in half. Set aside.

Peel the papaya and cut in half. Remove the seeds and dice into small pieces. Set aside.

Peel the banana and cut into chunks. Set aside.

Wash the cucumber and cut into thin slices. Fill the measuring cup and reserve the rest for later. Set aside.

Now, combine kiwis, papaya, basil, banana, and cucumber in a juicer and process until juiced. Transfer to a serving glass and add some ice before serving.

Enjoy!

Nutritional information per serving: Kcal: 365, Protein: 6.5g, Carbs: 107g, Fats: 2.8g

52.   Pepper Broccoli Juice

Ingredients:

1 large red bell pepper, chopped

1 cup of broccoli, chopped

1 cup of cucumber, sliced

1 large celery stalk, chopped

¼ tsp of ginger, ground

Preparation:

Wash the pepper and cut in half. Remove the seeds and stem. Cut into thin slices and set aside.

Wash the broccoli and trim off the outer wilted layers. Cut into small pieces and set aside.

Wash the cucumber and cut into thin slices. Fill the measuring cup and reserve the rest in the refrigerator.

Wash the celery stalk and cut into small pieces. Set aside.

Now, combine pepper, broccoli, cucumber, and celery in a juicer and process until well juiced. Transfer to a serving glass and stir in the ginger.

Refrigerate for 10 minutes before serving.

Nutritional information per serving: Kcal: 71, Protein: 4.9g, Carbs: 19.7g, Fats: 1g

53.   Raspberry Carrot Juice

Ingredients:

1 cup of raspberries

2 large carrots, peeled and chopped

1 large orange, wedged

¼ tsp of ginger, ground

1 tbsp of liquid honey

Preparation:

Using a colander, rinse the raspberries under cold running water and drain. Set aside.

Wash the carrots and peel them. Cut into small chunks and set aside.

Peel the orange and divide into wedges. Set aside.

Now, combine raspberries, carrots, and orange in a juicer and process until well juiced. Transfer to a serving glass and stir in the ginger and honey.

Refrigerate for 15 minutes before serving.

ADDITIONAL TITLES FROM THIS AUTHOR

70 Effective Meal Recipes to Prevent and Solve Being Overweight: Burn Fat Fast by Using Proper Dieting and Smart Nutrition

By Joe Correa CSN

48 Acne Solving Meal Recipes: The Fast and Natural Path to Fixing Your Acne Problems in Less Than 10 Days!

By Joe Correa CSN

41 Alzheimer's Preventing Meal Recipes: Reduce or Eliminate Your Alzheimer's Condition in 30 Days or Less!

By Joe Correa CSN

70 Effective Breast Cancer Meal Recipes: Prevent and Fight Breast Cancer with Smart Nutrition and Powerful Foods

By Joe Correa CSN

www.ingramcontent.com/pod-product-compliance
Lightning Source LLC
Chambersburg PA
CBHW030256030426
42336CB00009B/409